# YOUNGER FOR LIFE DIET Recipes

Delicious Recipes To Help You Look Great and Feel Your Best

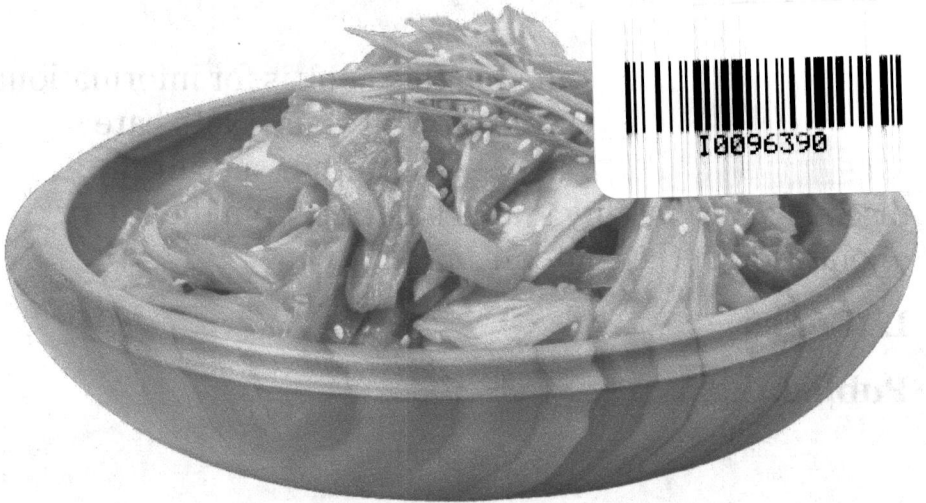

## Katherine Miller

**Disclaimer:**

The information provided in this book is for informational purposes only. Please consult with your health care provider for medical advice. The author specifically disclaims any liability that is incurred from the use or application of the contents of this book

**LitBooks**

**Publishing**

# Table of Contents

# Introduction

Welcome to a journey of discovery, where we explore the powerful connection between what we eat and how we feel. Picture this: I often get a knowing chuckle from audiences when I quip, "Depression isn't a Prozac deficiency." This humorous observation touches a deeper truth, resonating with a simple yet profound understanding – our health is not reliant on a deficit of pharmaceuticals. Imagine heart disease not as a lack of Lipitor, but as a signal of what our diets lack – the essential vitamins, minerals, phytochemicals, flavonoids, phenols, and the balance of fiber, protein, fat, and carbohydrates that keep our bodies humming with vitality for years.

I frequently encourage my listeners, "Nourish your body with what it needs, and it will reciprocate with vigor and wellness." This book is not just a collection of recipes; it's a manifesto that embraces the philosophy that while food may not be a panacea for all ailments, a thoughtful diet can be a formidable shield against many age-related diseases. Even if food cannot entirely cure an illness, it can undoubtedly alleviate its intensity, reduce its duration, and enhance overall health in the process.

Remember Hippocrates, the pioneer of modern medicine? He famously said, "Let food be thy medicine and medicine be thy food." This ancient wisdom aligns perfectly with his other guiding principle, "First do no harm." The culinary treasures and dietary guidelines in this book are a testament to these timeless words. Rest assured, nothing here will cause harm. Instead, I promise that every recipe and eating tip will supercharge your body – think of it as filling a Ferrari with premium fuel. This is your guide to optimal performance, a vibrant life, and endless energy, embracing the art of autojuvenation – where the right food choices can keep you youthful and spirited for decades to come. Let's embark on this exciting and transformative culinary adventure together!

# The Four Horsemen of Aging

"The Four Horsemen of Aging" is a critical topic in this book "Younger for Life Diet Recipes" Here we explore four fundamental processes that significantly influence the aging process. These processes can be directly linked to diseases commonly associated with aging, exacerbating their severity or complicating their treatment. The focus here is on how food can be used as a tool to combat these detrimental processes.

1. **The 1st Horseman of aging is Oxidative Damage:** This is a process you've likely witnessed in everyday life, such as when metal rusts or an apple slice turns brown. This damage is caused by free radicals, rogue oxygen molecules that cause similar harm to your cells and DNA. This oxidative stress accelerates aging, both internally and externally, evident in aging skin. The antidote? Antioxidants. They come in various forms, including vitamins C and E, minerals like zinc and selenium, and pigments like anthocyanins in blueberries and raspberries. Astaxanthin, the compound that gives wild salmon its pink color, is another potent antioxidant. The recipes in this book are rich

in these and many other antioxidants, offering a delicious way to combat oxidative damage.

2. **The 2nd Houseman of Aging is Inflammation:** Unlike the noticeable swelling from an injury, chronic inflammation is a silent process that damages the body's vascular system and can lead to heart attacks and strokes. It also harms brain cells, contributing to memory loss and diseases like Alzheimer's, and weakens the immune system. Combatting chronic inflammation starts with diet. Foods rich in natural anti-inflammatory compounds, such as quercetin found in apples and onions, resveratrol in dark grape skins, and omega-3 fatty acids in cold-water fish and flaxseed, are essential. The recipes presented are not only delicious but are specifically designed to be rich in compounds that mitigate inflammation, addressing the root cause of many age-related diseases.

3. **Glycation:** The Third Horseman of Aging is glycation, a process that occurs when excess sugar in the bloodstream binds to proteins, creating sticky, sugar-coated proteins. These glycosylated proteins can disrupt normal

bodily functions, leading to issues like circulatory complications, kidney problems, and vision impairments. This highlights the dangers of a diet high in sugar and processed carbohydrates, which not only spike blood sugar but also trigger an overproduction of insulin. Known as the "hunger hormone" and "fat storage hormone," insulin when chronically elevated, can increase blood pressure, promote weight gain, and contribute to a myriad of health issues. In this book, recipes are intentionally low in sugar and processed carbs to avoid these effects. When sweeteners are used, they're applied sparingly and always in combination with whole, nutritious foods. The desserts you'll find here are not only scrumptious but also contribute positively to your journey towards "Younger for Life," enhancing rather than detracting from your longevity.

4. **Stress:** The Fourth Horseman of Aging is stress. Although not directly combatted with food, stress, which has a significant hormonal component, is influenced by diet. Various factors, including dietary choices, can act as stressors, depleting essential nutrients like

vitamin B5 and vitamin C. Cortisol, the primary stress hormone, has a complex relationship with insulin. What you eat can indirectly affect stress levels, as well as provide comfort and familiarity, often why we turn to certain foods for solace. The key lies not in eliminating comfort foods, but in reinventing them in ways that contribute to longevity. This is elegantly achieved in the following recipes, where traditional dishes are reimagined with healthier ingredients without sacrificing taste. For example, a redefined "chicken parmigiana" uses whole-grain breadcrumbs and tofu to boost fiber and protein while keeping calories and fat low. Spaghetti squash substitutes traditional pasta for a lower glycemic impact and more nutrients. Likewise, a revamped mac and cheese incorporates whole-grain pasta, flaxseed, and butternut squash, lightening the calorie load while enriching nutrient content.

Every recipe in this book is in line with the younger for life Lifestyle Diet , blending the art of delicious cooking with the science of autojuvenation. By addressing these four critical processes, the culinary journey within these pages offers not just delightful flavors but a pathway to living "Younger for Life," harmonizing taste with timeless vitality.

# AutoJuvenation

In the pursuit of "Younger for Life," understanding the relationship between autojuvenation and the Four Horsemen of Aging offers a transformative insight into how we can harness the power of our diet to combat the inevitable process of aging. Autojuvenation, the concept of naturally rejuvenating the body, becomes a guiding principle in mitigating the detrimental effects of the Four Horsemen – oxidative damage, inflammation, glycation, and stress.

Dr. Anthony Youn, a renowned plastic surgeon, eloquently captures the essence of this relationship: "Aging might be a fact of life, but how we age is something we have considerable control over. The key is to understand the internal mechanisms that accelerate aging and counteract them with what we put on our plates. It's about embracing a lifestyle that turns back the clock from the inside out."

1. **Combatting Oxidative Damage:** Oxidative damage is akin to internal rusting, where free radicals wreak havoc on our cells. In autojuvenation, antioxidants in our diet act like a protective shield, neutralizing these harmful molecules. Dr. Youn often quotes,

"Think of antioxidants as your body's own team of superheroes, fighting the villainous free radicals and keeping you looking and feeling younger."

2. **Reducing Inflammation:** Inflammation is a silent saboteur, gradually impairing our body's functions. The anti-inflammatory foods play a vital role in autojuvenation. As Dr. Youn puts it, "Taming the flames of inflammation with your diet is like soothing a raging fire within. It's not just about feeling better, it's about giving your body a fighting chance against aging."

3. **Preventing Glycation:** Glycation, caused by excess sugar, leads to the stiffening and aging of tissues. In the context of autojuvenation, limiting sugar and processed carbs is like avoiding the glue that can gum up the body's works. Dr. Youn often remarks, "Cutting down on sugar isn't just about sweet restraint; it's about keeping your body's machinery running smoothly and youthfully."

4. **Managing Stress:** Though not directly linked to diet, stress influences and is

influenced by our nutritional choices. In autojuvenation, choosing foods that support hormonal balance and provide comfort can indirectly mitigate stress's aging effects. Dr. Youn notes, "Food can be both a source of comfort and a tool for combating stress. It's about finding that balance where what you eat nourishes both your body and soul."

By understanding and addressing these four key processes through the lens of autojuvenation, we can actively participate in the "Younger for Life" philosophy. It's not merely about adding years to life, but more importantly, adding life to those years. As Dr. Youn often states, "The secret to youth isn't found in a bottle or a surgery; it's on your plate. It's about making choices every day that rejuvenate and revitalize you from the inside out."

This holistic approach, blending the art of nourishment with the science of aging, is a testament to the power of food as a tool for transformation. It's an invitation to embark on a culinary journey that not only tantalizes the taste buds but also rejuvenates the body, embodying the essence of autojuvenation and leading us gracefully into a life that is indeed **"Younger for Life."**

# Why You Need This Cookbook To Stay Younger For Life

As we delve into the pages of this cookbook, we're not just exploring a collection of recipes; we're embarking on a transformative journey towards "Younger for Life." This cookbook is your essential guide, a treasure trove of culinary secrets that aligns perfectly with the principles of autojuvenation, providing you with the tools you need to combat the Four Horsemen of Aging.

Rest assured, every recipe within these pages has been carefully crafted to support your journey to a more youthful, vibrant self. This isn't just about tantalizing your taste buds – though it certainly will – it's about nourishing your body with the exact nutrients it needs to slow down the aging process and rejuvenate from within.

One of the cornerstones of this cookbook is its focus on anti-inflammatory foods. Chronic inflammation, as we've learned, is a silent yet potent ager of the body. The recipes here are rich in ingredients known for their inflammation-taming properties – foods that are not only delicious but also act as natural healers, working quietly and effectively to keep your body in a state of youthful equilibrium.

But the benefits don't stop there. This cookbook goes beyond just anti-inflammatory foods. It addresses each aspect of the Four Horsemen:

Antioxidant-Rich Foods: Bursting with ingredients high in essential antioxidants, these recipes combat oxidative damage, providing your cells with the defense they need against the free radicals that accelerate aging.

Low Glycemic Options: With a keen focus on low sugar and low processed carbohydrate choices, the recipes help prevent glycation, ensuring your tissues remain supple and youthful.

Stress-Reducing Meals: While food cannot eliminate stress, the choices made in these recipes support hormonal balance and provide a comforting, nurturing experience, contributing to overall stress reduction.

In "Younger for Life," every recipe is an invitation to a healthier, more youthful you. This cookbook isn't just a compilation of meals; it's a blueprint for a lifestyle that embraces the art of eating well to age well. With each dish, you're not only enjoying a delicious meal but also investing in your longevity, ensuring that each year added to your life is full of health, vitality, and youthfulness.

So, whether you're flipping through these pages to find a soothing, anti-inflammatory soup, a rejuvenating antioxidant-rich salad, or a comforting, low-glycemic dessert, know that you're taking a step towards embracing a "Younger for Life" philosophy. This cookbook is more than just a companion in your kitchen; it's a guide on your journey to autojuvenation, a journey where every meal brings you closer to a life of vibrant health and youthful energy.

# 101 Approved Younger For Life Recipes

## Blueberry-Pie Smoothie
### Ingredients

- One burro banana

- One teaspoon Bromide Plus Powder

- 1/4 cup cooked amaranth

- One tablespoon homemade walnut butter

- 2 cups homemade soft-jelly coconut milk

- Two tablespoons date sugar

- 1 cup fresh blueberries

### Preparations

Put all ingredients in a high-speed blender and blend. Keep smoothie in the freezer and drink when cold.

## Alkaline-Electric Spring Salad
### Ingredients

- 1 cup cherry tomatoes

- 4 cups seasonal approved greens of your choice (watercress, dandelion greens, wild arugula)

- 1/4 cup approved herbs of your choice

- 1/4 cup walnuts

<u>Ingredients for the dressing</u>

- 3-4 key limes

- Sea salt and cayenne pepper, to taste

- 1 tablespoon of homemade raw sesame "tahini" butter

<u>Preparations</u>

Juice the limes, beat the lime juice with the homemade "tahini" oil. Add cayenne pepper and seal salt. Divide the cherry tomatoes, add veggies, cherry tomatoes, and herbs to a big bowl. Use your hand to massage this mixture. Add more salt, herbs, and cayenne pepper if you like. Enjoy.

## The Kidney Cleanse Juice
<u>Ingredients</u>

1-2 cups of soft-jelly coconut water

4 seeded cucumbers

2-3 key limes

1 bunch basil or sweet basil leaves

1/2 tsp. Bromide Plus Powder

## Preparations

Blend the basil, cucumber, basil, and key lime. Serve juice with bromide plus powder and coconut water. Mix well and drink.

# Fabulous Hydration Smoothie
## Ingredients

•1/2 cup raspberries

•1 cup watermelon

•1/4 seeded cucumber

•1/2 cup soft-jelly coconut water

•1 juiced key lime

## Preparations

Peel and main the cucumber. Cut into tiny bits. Put all the ingredients in a high-speed blender and blend. Allow to calm down before drinking.

# Immunity-Boosting Smoothie

## Ingredients

- 1 Seville orange

- 1/2 mango

- 1 cup brewed Dr. Sebi's Immune Support Herbal Tea

- 1 tablespoon date sugar or agave syrup

- 1 tablespoon coconut oil

- 1 key juice lime

## Preparations

Boil two cups of water purified and add a cube of Dr. Sebi's Immune Help Herbal Tea. Boil for 15 minutes. Let it cool. Cut the mango into bits and peel the orange Seville, put it into a high-speed mixer, add other ingredients, and blend. Enjoy!

# Creamy Relaxing Smoothie

## Ingredients

- 1 Burro banana

- 1/2 cup prepared Dr. Sebi's Nerve/Stress Relief Herbal Tea

- 1/4 avocado

- 1 cup soft-jelly coconut milk

- 1/4 seeded cucumber

- 1 tablespoon chopped walnuts

- 1 tablespoon date sugar or agave syrup (optional)

## Preparations

Boil 2 cups of refined water and add 1 table cube of Dr. Sebi's Nerve/Stress Relief Herbal Tea. Steep for about 15 minutes and allow to cool. Mix half a cup of tea with other ingredients and put it in a high-speed blender.

## Nori-Burritos

## Ingredients

- 450 gr. Seeded cucumber

- 4 sheets nori seaweed

- A handful of amaranth or dandelion greens

- 1 small zucchini

- A handful of sprouted hemp seeds

- 1/2 ripe mango

- 1 tbs. tahini

- 1 ripe avocado

- Sesame seeds to taste

## Preparations

Put the Nori sheet on a cutting board. Place all the ingredients on the nori sheet and leave a large margin of visible nori to the right.

With both hands, fold the sheet of nori from the edge to edge unto of the fillings. Divide into thick slices and sprinkle with seeds of sesame.

## Younger For Life Orange Creamsicle Smoothie

### Ingredients

- 1/2 Burro banana

- 3 peeled Seville oranges

- 1 cup of coconut water

- 1/2 tsp. Bromide Plus Powder

- Date sugar to taste

## Preparations

Fill in all ingredients and blend until a fine blend. Serve and enjoy.

## Green Detox Smoothie
### Ingredients

- 1 cup Romaine lettuce

- 1/2 burro banana

- 2 – 3 tbsp. key lime juice

- 1/4 cup blueberries

- 1/2 cup ginger tea

- 1/2 cup soft jelly coconut water

### Preparations

Prepare tea and allow cool. Blend entire ingredients and enjoy.

## Detox Berry Smoothie
### Ingredients

- ¼ Avocado

- 1 medium-size Burro Banana

- 1 cup of Berries (a mix of blue, rasp, and strawberries or just blueberries)

- 2 cups of fresh Lettuce

- 1 fruit Seville Orange

- 2 Cups of Water

- 1 tablespoon of Hemp Seeds

## Preparations

Add some water into blended, then add veggies and fruits.

Blend them all until smooth. Enjoy.


## Spelt French Toast
## Ingredients

- 2 tsp. of maple crystals

- 2 tsp. of Quinoa flakes

- 1 cup of Almond Milk

- 1/2 tsp. of sea salt

• 2 slices of Spelt Bread

• 2 tsp. of spelt flour

Preparations

Put all the ingredients in a bowl. Lower the bread into the mixture and well soaked but not soggy. Get a pan heated with olive oil and fry both sides gently.

## Kamut Raisin Pancakes
### Ingredients

2 cups of Kamut flour

1 2/3 tsp. of seams powder

1/4 cup of raisins

2 tsp. of vanilla extract

1 1/2 cup of almond milk

1 cup of maple crystals

Preparations

Put the Kamut flour and powdered sea moss in a pan. Put the raisins, maple crystals, and vanilla extract inside. Add the almond milk as well. Pour into a hot skillet and cook both sides till done.

# Kamut Puff Cereal
## Ingredients

- 1/4 cup of chopped dates

- 1 cup of Kamut puffs

- 1/4 cup of chopped almonds

- 1 cup of hot Almond milk

- 1/4 of raisins

- 1/4 cup of agave nectar

## Preparations

Get a bowl, mix the almonds, cereal, dates, and agave nectar. Add the almond milk. Enjoy your meal.

# Sea moss Breakfast Shake
## Ingredients

- 1 tsp. of sea moss

- 3-4 cups of water

- 4 bp of almond butter

- 2 tsp. of cinnamon

- 3 cups of almond milk

- 1 3 tsp. of vanilla extract

- cup of maple syrup

## Preparations

Get some hot water and put the stems inside. Add the cinnamon, maple syrup, vanilla extract, almond butter, and almond milk. Blend this mix until a fine blend. Chill and serve.

## Papaya Breakfast Shake

### Ingredients

1 tsp. of seams

1/2 cup of fresh or frozen papaya

1/2 cup of agave nectar

1/2 cup of cold water

2 cups of almond milk

### Preparations

Get the sea moss and blend with water. Add papaya, milk, and agave nectar. Blend till smooth and then keep in the refrigerator, serve cold.

# Spelt Strawberry Waffles
## Ingredients

2 cups of spelt flour

6 strawberries cut into small pieces

1/4 cup of agave nectar

1 tsp. of vanilla extract

1 tsp. of seams

1/2 cup of almond milk

1/4 cup of water

## Preparations

Add bits of strawberry, seams, and spelt flour. Add vanilla extract, water, almond milk, and agave nectar. Blend and then add to the waffle machine and cook.

# Cream of Kamut
## Ingredients

•1 cup of maple crystals

•1 tsp. of cinnamon

•1 1/2 tsp. of vanilla extract

- 2 cups of water

- 1 1/2 cup of Kamut flour

- 4 cups of almond milk

Preparations

Put water in a pot to boil. When boiled, turn off. Put the Kamut flour till it is thick. Add the cinnamon, vanilla extract, almond milk, and maple crystals. Stir, serve and enjoy.

# Cream of Rye

## Ingredients

- 1 tsp. of vanilla extract

- 1/4 cup of agave nectar

- 1/2 cup of almond milk

- 1 1/2 cup of cream of rye

- 1/2 cup of water

## Preparations

Boil water in a kettle. When water boils, turn off the heat.

Pour the water into a pot, put the rye cream mix into it till it gets thick. Add the milk, vanilla extract, and agave nectar. Stir, serve and enjoy.

# Blueberry Spelt Muffins

## Ingredients

- 1 cup of almond milk

- 1/2 cup of sea moss

- 1/2 cup of sea moss

- 3/4 cup of spelt flour

- 1 tsp. of baking powder

- 1/3 cup of maple syrup

- 3/4 cup of Kamut flour

- 1/4 tsp. of sea salt

- 1 cup of blueberries

## Preparations

Heat your oven to 400F. Place your baking cups inside the muffin pan. Get a mixing dish and put your flour, baking powder, salt, sea moss, and syrup and mix. Add almond milk and mix properly. Wray the blueberries in it.

Pour into baking cups to bake for 30 mins.

## Younger For Life Sleepy Time drink
## Ingredients

- ¼ Cup of cooked Quinoa

- 2 cups of Amaranth Greens

- ½ Cup of Dr. Sebi's Nerve Relief Herbal Tea

- ½ Cup of Dr. Sebi's Stomach Relief Herbal Tea

- A lump of Burro Banana

- ¼ Cup of Cherries

- Agave syrup to taste

## Preparation

Make the nerve relief and stomach relief tea as specified on the pack. Put water into a blender, add all ingredients ad blend well till a fine blend. Put into a cup and enjoy.

## Vegetable Mushroom Soup

### Ingredients

- 1 small red and green bell pepper chopped

- 1 cup quinoa

- 1 clove

- 2 large peeled and chopped chayote squash

- 2-3 bunches of kale

- Springwater

- 2 onions chopped finely

- 1/2 lb. Kamut spiral pasta

- 1 bunch spinach, washed and steamed

- 2 tbsp. olive oil

- 1/2 tsp. of marjoram, rosemary, thyme, red pepper, oregano, and cumin

- 1 chopped lb. oyster mushrooms

## Preparations

Take a saucepan and add olive oil and heat up. Sauté the onions, mushrooms, and bell peppers. Take a soup pot, add the mushroom with spring water. Put in the chayote squash, oregano, marjoram, garlic, thyme, red pepper, cumin, and quinoa. Allow to simmer for 45 mins then put Kamut pasta to simmer for another 15 mins.

Then add the spinach and stir. Serve when soft.

## Pasta Salad
### Ingredients

- 1/2 cup of olive oil

- 3-4 dashes of cilantro

- 4 tbs. of sea salt

- 1/4 cup of almond milk

- 1/2 cup of chopped onions

- 3 tbs. of maple syrup

- 1/4 cup of fresh lime juice

- 1 1/2 cup of sun-dried tomatoes

- 2 avocados cut into small pieces

- 2 boxes of spelt penne

## Preparations

Cook the pasta. Add all the ingredients into a large bowl, turn all ingredients until well mixed.

## Vegetable Patties
### Ingredients

- 1 pinch of African red pepper

- 3 tbsp. olive oil

- 1 medium yellow onion chopped well

- Spring Water

- 1 bunch of kale greens cut fine

- 1/2 red and green peppers chopped

- 1/4 cup sea moss powder

- 2 chayote squash diced

- Kamut Flour

- 1 bunch of broccoli chopped well

## Preparations

Place a skillet on heat and heat up putting 3 three tbsp. of olive oil. Add onions, African red pepper, chayote squash, bell pepper, and ground cumin and fry for 3 mins. Simmer the kale and broccoli for 12 mins.

## Preparations for making of flour of Kamut

Mix sea moss with flour and water. Roll on a floured surface divided into circles of 10" diameter. Put cooked veggies in half a circle. Cover the veggies by folding the other half over them. Use a fork to pinch the edges to close.

Place patties and bake until golden brown.

## Mushroom Patties
### Ingredients

- 1/4 cup of spelt flour

- 4 tbsp. sea salt

- 1/4 bunch of cilantro

- 1/2 cup bell peppers

- 2 portabella mushrooms

- 2 tsp. onion powder

- 1 tsp. dill

- 1/4 tsp. oregano

- 1 Pinch of cayenne pepper

<u>Preparations</u>

Soak mushrooms in cold water for 1 minute. Drain water and put the mushroom in a food processor with scallions and bell peppers. Add cilantro, flour, and the seasoning of your choice. Blend properly and shape the pastries. Add 2 tbsp. of olive oil to a heated pan, cook the pastries on both sides till done.

## The Greatest Greens
<u>Ingredients</u>

- 1 tsp. of cayenne or chili powder

- 3 tbsp. sea salt

- 1/4 cup olive oil

- 3 packs of mustard and turnips green 1/2 of each

- 2 cups of chopped onions

## Preparations

Heat your skillet, add onions and cook till golden brown. Add your greens and simmer for 20 mins. Season with ground cayenne and sea salt.

## Veggies Stir Fry Medley
### Ingredients

- 3 tbsp. olive oil

- 8 chopped cherry tomatoes

- 1 small chopped red and green pepper

- 1 cup of chopped broccoli

- 1/2 chopped small yellow onion

- 2 sliced zucchini

- 1 pkg. sliced oyster mushrooms

## Preparations

Place olive oil in a hot skillet and add tomatoes and onions. Put seasoning as desired and sauté for about 3-4 minutes. Toss in your mushrooms and fry for 4 more mins. Then add zucchini, bell peppers, and broccoli and fry for another 4 mins. Your food is ready.

## Stuffed Bell Peppers
## Ingredients

•1/2 tsp. sweet basil

•3 tbsp. olive oil

•1/2 tsp. sea salt

•1/2 tsp. dill

•1/4 tsp. of ground cumin

•1/2 red bell peppers chopped well

•2 slices of crumbled Kamut or spelt bread toasted

•1 1/2 cup of quinoa

•2 green bell peppers

•1 lb. oyster or brown button mushroom

## Preparations

Steam your bell peppers till they are soft. Over low heat, take your pan and add some water, put in the quinoa grain, and cover the pan. Cook till the quinoa has taken all the water and set aside.

Sauté red bell peppers and mushrooms in olive oil. Add your spices and more olive oil to the bell peppers. Mix the remaining seasoning with the quinoa, mushrooms, and red bell pepper. Fill up the mix within the bell peppers, spread the bread crumbs over it. Bake at 250 degrees for about 15 minutes in a heated oven. Serve hot with a green leafy salad.

## Wild Rice
### Ingredients

- 1/8 tsp. African red pepper

- 1 tsp. sea salt

- 2 tsp. oregano

- 1 tsp. thyme

- 1/8 cup olive oil

- 1 cup mushrooms, chopped medium, fine (oyster or brown button)

- 1 small red pepper

- 1 medium yellow onion chopped fine

- Springwater

- Wild rice

## Preparations

Soak rice in spring water overnight or cook the rice and set aside. Take a saucepan and pour olive oil in. Sauté the vegetables and mushrooms for 3 mins. Put in thyme, red pepper, oregano, and sea salt. Fold in the cooked rice and cook for another 20 mins.

## Tomato Sauce Spaghetti Recipe
## Ingredients

- Vita Spelt Pasta

- 1/2 cup of olive oil

- 2 cups of tomato sauce

- 4 tbsp. of sea salt

- 1 1/2 tbsp. of onion powder

- 2 tbsp. of cayenne/chili powder

•3 tbsp. of maple syrup

## Preparations

Cook pasta and strain when cooked. In another pot, add olive oil, tomato sauce, onion powder, cayenne/chili powder, sea salt, and maple syrup and cook for 10 mins. Add pasta to the sauce and let cook for 5 mins. Food is ready, serve and enjoy.

## Lasagna Special
## Ingredients

•Almond cheddar cheese

•8 fresh tomatoes

•Sea salt

•Oregano

•2 lb., mushrooms

•Spelt lasagna pasta

•1 chopped yellow onion

•1 chopped red bell pepper

•Crumbled Bay leaf

•2 tbsp. olive oil

## Preparations of Tomato sauce

Heat the pan and apply olive oil to it. Add onions, oregano, bell peppers, bay leaf, and salt and sauté. Boil your tomatoes for 10 minutes. Put in ice water for 5 mins, rinse, and peel the skin off the tomatoes.

Blend tomatoes in a blender to make fresh tomato sauce. Take a pan and add tomato sauce and sauté, simmer for about 45 min. Divide the sauce into two for a mushroom sauce later, and the other half will go for layering.

8. Put aside half of the sauce that will be used to produce a

## Preparations of Mushroom sauce

Put mushrooms in some water, soak for 1 minute, strain and slice. Place in 1/2 of the saved sauce, keep aside for layering, and season to taste sauté for about 2 minutes.

## Preparation of Pasta

Cook pasta as directed and drain when done under cold water. Place a baking dish and put in tomato sauce and put a pasta layer over it, then mushroom sauce layer over that. Add a layer of cheddar almond. Repeat this procedure until the dish is almost full. Put the leftover almond cheddar on top of 2 cups of sauce and cook for 20 minutes in a 350-degree oven before the almond cheddar is smelted.

## Hot Veggie Wraps
### Ingredients

• 1 cup of diced bell peppers

• 2 cups onion

• 1/2 cup of mushrooms chopped

• 3 cups diced tomatoes

### Preparations

Fry all the veggies for 5 minutes, and then stir. Warm up the spelt tortilla. Put the fried veggies in and enjoy.

## Taquitos
### Ingredients

4 cups of chopped mushrooms

2 cups of chopped onion

2 tbsp. oregano

2 tbsp. tomato sauce

2 tsp. ground thyme

2 tsp. onion powder

3 tbsp. sea salt

2 tsp. chili powder

Preparations

1/4 cup olive oil to the mixing pan. Toss in the onion and sauté till golden brown. Add seasoning and tightly bundle the corn shells into it. Then fry until mildly crunchy.

## Mushroom Salad
Ingredients

- 1/2 tsp. dill

- 1/4 cup fresh lime juice

- 1/2 tsp. sea salt

- 1/2 tsp. basil

- 1/2 cup olive oil

- 1 sm. Diced red onion

- 1/4 bunch of torn romaine lettuce

- 1/4 bunch or torn red leaf lettuce

- 1/2 chopped red bell pepper

- 1/2 lb. fresh mushrooms

- 1/4 bunch of torn fresh spinach

Preparations

Wash the mushrooms well, dry them, and have them cut. Add in your lime juice, dill, bell pepper, onion, basil, olive oil, and sea salt to taste. Marinade in the fridge for half an hour. Wash the greens properly, dry, and cut. Put the greens with the mushrooms and blend well. Enjoy!

## Avocado Dressing
Ingredients

- 1/2 small red onion

- 3 Ripe avocados, peeled and seeded

- 1/4 tsp. sea salt

- 1/2 tsp. thyme

- 1 tsp. cumin

- 1 tsp. oregano

- 1/2 tsp. sweet basil

- 1/2 tsp. sweet basil

- 1 tsp. chili powder

- Few sprigs of cilantro

- 1/4 cup fresh lime juice

- 1/2 tomato peeled

- Pinch Cayenne Pepper

- 4 tbsp. pure olive oil

## Preparations

Add avocado to the food processor to make a puree of it. Add the ingredients and 2 teaspoons of spring water and mix well. Blend gently and pour over the salad. Season to your desired taste.

## Vegetable Salad
### Ingredients

1/4 tsp. cumin

1/2 tsp. dill

1/2 bunch of chopped cilantro

Sweet basil to taste

1/2 cup olive oil

1/4 cup fresh lime juice

1/2 bunch of torn watercress

1/2 bunch of torn romaine lettuce

1/2 lb. fresh string beans

Preparations

Add some olive oil to a pan and add dill, cumin, basil, and lime juice when heated up. Marinade in the refrigerator for about 2 hours. Mix well with lettuce, watercress, and cilantro. Enjoy.

## Lime and Olive Oil Dressing
Ingredients

1/4 tsp. ground cumin

1/4 tsp. oregano

1/8 cup spring water

1/2 cup olive oil

1/4 freshly squeeze lime juice

1/4 tsp. thyme

1/4 tsp. sweet basil

1 tbs. maple syrup

## Preparations

Get a glass bottle and place in all the ingredients. Shake the container gently. Enjoy.

# Creamy Salad Dressing

## Ingredients

1/4 tsp. sea salt

1 tsp. maple syrup

1/4 tsp. thyme

1/2 tsp. sweet basil

1/2 cup fresh lime juice

1/4 tsp. ground cumin

2 green onions

4 tbs. almond butter

## Preparations

Place all the condiments inside a glass container and 2 teaspoons of spring water. Shake it slightly and enjoy.

# Tamarind Water
## Ingredients

100g tamarind pulp

2 liters fresh spring water

Agave syrup or date sugar

600ml boiling spring water

<u>Preparations</u>

Boil some water and pour it on the tamarind pulp, leave for 20 mins to soak. Break the pulp with a knife, use a strainer to drain paste into a bowl. Use a spoon to push all the pulp you possibly can take out and scrape any tamarind puree into the bowl from under the strainer. Take some spring water and blend the liquid. Sweeten with agave syrup or date sugar.

## Cucumber Dressing

<u>Ingredients</u>

1/2 tsp. thyme

1/4 cup of finely chopped green onions

1/4 cup fresh lime juice

Few sprigs of chopped cilantro

1-1/2 cup spring water

1/4 tsp. dill

4 tbs. pure olive oil

10 almonds, raw, unsalted

1/2 tsp. sea salt

3 med. Peeled cucumbers

## Preparations

Blend 10 almonds in spring water in a high-speed processor for about 2 mins. Strain liquid and set aside.

Puree cucumbers and almonds in a processor/blender. Add some lime juice and all the ingredients. Blend them lightly and pour your salad over it and enjoy.

## Xave's Delight
## Ingredients

- 1 oz spring water

- 3 oz. sesame tahini

- 1/2 tsp. red pepper

- 1 tsp. sea salt

- 3 tbs. maple syrup

- 2 fresh limes squeezed

## Preparations

Get a glass bottle and add some spring water, maple syrup, sesame tahini, two limes, red pepper, and sea salt. Shake and use for your salad dressing.

## Tamarind Paste
### Ingredients

250 gr of natural tamarind

3 cups of spring water

### Preparations

Clean the tamarind and take out the skin, seeds, or particles. Dip tamarind in two cups of hot water till tamarind gets soft. When soft, blend till a fine blend using a high-speed processor. Sift it and trash the debris. Take the pulp and simmer over medium heat for about 5 mins. Take an airtight container and pour the paste when it has cooled down.

## Quinoa Bread
### Ingredients

60 ml (2 fly oz / ¼ cup) grapeseed oil

1/2 cup water

1/2 of juiced key lime

1/2 teaspoon sea salt

300 g (10 ½ oz or 1 3/4 cups) whole uncooked quinoa seed

Preparations

Dip quinoa in a lot of cold water and put it in the refrigerator all through the night. Heat up the oven to 160 C / 320 F. strain the quinoa and then wash into a sieve. Take out all the liquid from the quinoa and blend. Add grape-seed oil and half a cup of water, lime juice, and sea salt and mix. Blend with a food processor for 3 mins.

A batter consistency with some whole quinoa already left in the mix could imitate the bread mix. Spoon on both sides and the foundation into a loaf tin lined with parchment paper. Bake till solid or when it bounces back when you push with your fingertips.

Take it out from the oven to cool in the pan for about 30 mins and remove from pan. Eat when cool.

## Plant-Based Quinoa Bowl
Ingredients

•1 Tablespoon of Grapeseed Oil

- 1 Handful of Approved Greens

- 1 Cup of Cooked Quinoa

- 2 Cups of Chopped Approved Vegetables

## Preparation

Put a tablespoon of grapeseed oil in a big pan and heat up. Sauté the diced vegetables till they are tender. Mix the cooked quinoa, vegetables, and fresh greens, season with cayenne pepper, and taste season with sea salt.

## Dr. Sebi's Mango Salad
### Ingredients

- Cayenne Pepper and Sea Salt

- ¼ Cup Cherry Tomatoes

- 2 Mangoes

- ¼ Red Onion

- ½ Seeded Cucumber

- ½ Green Bell Pepper

- 1 key Lime

## Preparation

Dice the mangoes, cut the cherry tomatoes into tiny cubes and chop the onions as well. Add the finely chopped bell peppers and seeded cucumber.

Mix well in a small bowl, add a squeeze of lime juice to the salad. Add pepper and salt to taste, leave to marinate in the fridge for about 20 minutes. Serve and enjoy.

## Basil Avocado Pasta Salad
### Ingredients

• ¼ Cup of Olive Oil

• 1 Tablespoon of Agave Syrup

• 1 Chopped Avocado 1 Cup of Chopped Fresh Basil

• 1 Tablespoon of Key Lime Juice

• 4 Cups of Cooked Spelt Pasta (used any of Dr. Sebi's approved pasta)

• 1 Pint of Cherry Tomatoes, Halved.

### Preparation

Put the already cooked pasta in a medium bowl. Add the avocado, basil, tomatoes and mix all the ingredients properly. Add a dash of lime, sea salt for taste, oil, and agave syrup in another bowl, and mix till a fine mixture. Pour this mixture on the set aside pasta and stir till well mixed.

## Kamut Breakfast Porridge
### Ingredients

•1 cup (7 ounces) of Kamut

•1 Tablespoon of Coconut Oil

•3¾ Cups of either Homemade Walnut Milk/Soft-Jelly Coconut milk

•4 Tablespoon of Agave Syrup

•½ Tablespoon of Sea Salt

### Preparation

Grind the Kamut and get about 1¼ cups of the milled Kamut.

Take a saucepan, add the walnut or coconut milk, sea salt, and the milled Kamut and mix well.

Leave it to boil on high heat for about 10 mins. Reduce from high to low and then simmer. Stir till you get the perfect consistency or thickness. Turn off the heat and add the coconut oil and the agave syrup and stir. You can choose to relish the meal with fresh fruits and enjoy.

# Stewed Okra & Tomatoes Wild Rice

## Ingredients

• Cayenne Pepper

• 2 Cups of Fresh Okra

• 1 Medium Onion

• ½ Cup of Fresh Spring Water

• 1 Tablespoon of Avocado Oil

• Sea Salt

• 1 Cup of Cherry Tomatoes

## Preparation

Prep the onions, dice till alongside the cherry tomatoes. Take your skillet and add avocado oil, when heated, add the diced onions. Stir-fry till translucent. When translucent, add the okra and spring water. Reduce the heat and cook for 10 minutes.

Add the chopped cherry tomatoes, leave the heat on low and cook till the okra is cooked well. Add sea salt for taste and pepper.

# Dandelion Strawberry Salad
## Ingredient

- 2 Tablespoon of Key Lime Juice

- 2 Tablespoon of Grapeseed Oil

- Sea Salt

- 1 Medium Red Onion (Sliced)

- 4 Cups Dandelion Greens

- 10 Ripe Strawberry (Sliced)

## Preparation

Take a nonstick frying pan and add the grapeseed oil. Heat the pan with the content and then add the chopped red onions and a pinch of the sea salt to taste. Stir occasionally till soft, light brown, and reduced in size.

In a small bowl, add the diced strawberry and 1 teaspoon of key lime juice and stir. Wash the dandelion greens and chop as preferred.

Add the leftover key lime juice to the pan if the onions are almost ready. Cook till thick and it covers the onions, then after about 2 mins, take the onions out of the pan.

Set aside the salad bowl that has the strawberries and other contents earlier mixed, add the onions and greens and do a thorough mix, add a dash of sea salt and mix in well.

## Green Detox Smoothie & Juicy Portobello Burger

### Ingredients

- ½ Cup of Soft Jelly Coconut Water

- ½ Burro Banana

- ¼ Cup of Blueberries

- ½ Cup Ginger Tea

- 1 Cup Romaine Lettuce

- 2 – 3 Tablespoon of Key Lime Juice

### Preparation

Make the tea and let it cool, then mix all the ingredients with a blender.

### Ingredient for Juicy Portobello Burger

- 1 Cup Purslane

- 2 Large Portobello Mushroom Caps

- 1 Tablespoon of Dried Oregano

- 1 Avocado (Sliced)

- 2 Tablespoon of Dried Basil

- 1 Tomato (Sliced)

- 3 Tablespoon of Olive Oil

## Preparation

Take off the stems of the mushroom, like about ½ the top of the mushroom. Get a small bowl and add the basil, onion powder, cayenne pepper, oregano, and olive oil, and mix properly. Grease the foil with grapeseed oil so the mushroom caps don't stick. After greasing the foil, add the mushroom.

Add the marinade on top of the mushroom with a spoon and let it settle for 10 mins. Heat the oven to 425 °F, then let the mushroom bake for another 10 mins. Check on your cooking to know how to read it is so you can flip it to the other side to cook for 10 mins more. When ready, serve with any toppings you choose and enjoy.

## Magic Green Falafel
### Ingredients

- 1 Large Onion (Chopped)

- 2 Cups of Dry Garbanzo Beans (Chickpeas)

- 2/3 Cup of Fresh Basil

- 1/2 Cup of Fresh Dill

- 1/3 Cup of Red Bell Pepper (Chopped)

- 1 teaspoon of Sea Salt

- 1/4 Teaspoon of Oregano

- 1/2 Cup of Garbanzo Bean Flour

- Grapeseed or Avocado Oil for Frying

Preparation

First, boil the chickpeas till soft. When tender drain and rinse your beans.

Put the chickpeas the rest of the ingredients in a food processor and pulse till a fine blend. Taste and add more seasoning if the need arises.

Scoop out the mix with your hands and put it in a bowl. Make small balls of the mix and wrap them inlined parchment paper. Keep in the refrigerator to cool for an hour. Fill a big skillet with oil and cook over low heat for 5 minutes and then fry the Magic Green Falafels for 3 minutes on both sides.

## Grilled Romaine Lettuce Salad

### Ingredients

•Cayenne Pepper

•1 Tablespoon of Key Lime Juice.

•1 Tablespoon of Fresh Basil (Chopped)

•1 Tablespoon of Agave Syrup

•1 Tablespoon of Red Onion (Finely Chopped)

•4 Tablespoons of Olive Oil

•Sea Salt to taste

•4 Small Heads Romaine Lettuce (Rinsed)

### Preparation

Cut the lettuce in halves and put it in a large nonstick pan.

Grill lettuce without oil, when both sides of the lettuce turn brown, take from the heat. Let the vegetables cool on a large tray.

Mix the fresh basil, agave syrup, red onion, olive oil, and key lime juice in a mixing bowl. Add pepper and salt and mix properly.

Transfer the sautéed lettuce into a serving dish, spread the dressing over it, and enjoy.

## Green Pancake
### Ingredients

•½ Cup of Spring Water

•¼ Cup of Blueberries

•1 Handful of Amaranth Green

•1 Tablespoon of Agave Syrup

•1 tablespoon of your favorite Nut Butter for more protein (Brazil nut butter, homemade tahini, or homemade walnut)

•½ Cup of Chickpea Flour

•½ Teaspoon of Sea Salt

### Preparation

Blend all the ingredients in a blender till smooth. Allow the mixture to rest for 10 minutes. Be careful with the water you add to the mix if not mixture may not cook well.

Heat a nonstick pan over low heat, scoop the blended mix in the shape of pancakes (the sizes are at your discretion) and allow to cook till they look fluffy and cooked properly on both sides. Serve on a plate, garnish with burro banana, blueberries, or agave syrup. Enjoy.

## Alkaline Mushroom Gravy

### Ingredients

• 2 Tablespoon of Grapeseed Oil

• 1 Cup of Thinly Sliced Mushroom (except for shiitake)

• 1 Pinch each of Cayenne pepper and Sea Salt

• 1½ Tablespoon of Amaranth or Spelt Flour

• ½ Teaspoon of Fresh Thyme

• ¼ of an Onion (Diced)

• ½ Cup of Homemade Approved Vegetable Broth

• 1 Cup of Homemade Walnut Milk

• 2 Tablespoons of Finely Cut Walnuts

## Preparation

Under medium heat, place a saucepan or a cast-iron skillet and add grapeseed oil. Allow to heat up and then add the onions, mushroom, and cayenne pepper, and salt as preferred. Allow cooking for 4 minutes. When the onions are translucent, add the amaranth and spelt flour and mix thoroughly and cook for about a minute.

Slowly mix the homemade vegetables broth and the walnut milk, half cup at a time. Then season with sea salt and cayenne pepper to taste. Cook till it gets thick, keep stirring under low heat. Feel free to add more seasoning if the taste is unsuitable.

Then add the walnuts, mix well and add more walnut milk till the consistency is as desired. Serve and enjoy with bread from any of Dr. Sebi's approved grains or a plant-based biscuit.

# Zucchini Bread Pancake

## Ingredients

- ½ Cup of Chopped Walnuts

- 2 Cups of Homemade Walnut Milk

- 2 Tablespoon of Date Sugar

- 1 Cup of Finely Shredded Zucchini

- 2 Cups of Spelt or Kamut Flour

- ¼ Cup of Mashed Burro Banana

## Preparation

Whisk the flour and date sugar in a large bowl. Add the crushed burro banana and the walnut milk and stir till a fine blend. Take a bowl, add walnuts and the shredded zucchini and mix well.

On medium heat, heat up the grapeseed oil in the skillet. Add the blend into the skillet in the shape of pancakes, cook both sides till properly cooked. Serve and joy with agave syrup.

# Zoodles with Avocado Pear

## Ingredients

- 2 Cups of Basil

- 2 Large Zucchinis

- ½ Cup of Walnuts

- 2 Avocados

- ½ Cup of Water

- 24 Sliced Cherry Tomatoes

- Sea Salt to taste

- 4 Tablespoons of Key Lime Juice

Preparation

Use a spiralizer or any other alternative at your disposal to make the zucchini noodles. Add all the ingredients aside from the cherry tomatoes into a blender and blend till smooth.

Put the cherry tomatoes, avocado sauce, and noodles in a bowl to mix. Well properly mixed, serve on a plate, and enjoy.

## Classic Household Hummus
Ingredients

- 1/3 Cup Homemade Tahini Butter

- 2 Tablespoons Olive Oil

- 2 Tablespoons Key Lime Juice

- A Dash of Onion Powder

- 1 Cup of Cooked Chickpeas

- Sea Salt to taste

Preparations

Put all the ingredients in an efficient blender and blend.

Serve and enjoy.

## Wild Rice Mushroom
Ingredients

- 3 Tablespoon of Grapeseed Oil

- 2 Six-Pound Packages Wild Rice and Long Grain Mix

- 1 Large diced Sweet Onion

- ½ Cup Marsala

- 12 Ounces of chopped Assorted Fresh Mushrooms

- ¼ Teaspoon Salt

- ½ Cup Chopped Fresh Flat-Leaf Parsley

## Preparation

First wash the rice properly, then per-boil the rice. Put a large skillet and add grapeseed oil and heat on low-medium heat. Add onions and sauté till brown.

Put in the mushroom, add salt for taste, and cook until the mushroom becomes soft. Put in the marsala and cook for 3 minutes.

Mix the mushroom with the parsley and add in the rice.

Serve and enjoy.

## Detox Salad Burritos & Detox Smoothie

### Ingredients

•4 Kamut Flour Tortillas

•2 Cups Wild Arugula or any of Dr. Sebi's approved grain

•1 Tablespoon of Key Lime Juice

•1 Cup of Cooked Chickpeas (Garbanzo Beans)

•1 Tablespoon of Homemade Raw Sesame Tahini Butter

•Cayenne Pepper

- 2 cups of Cherry Tomatoes

- Sea salt to taste

## Preparations

Get a cup, add the key lime juice with the raw sesame tahini butter, and mix. Then set it aside.

Mix the chickpeas, cherry tomatoes, and wild arugula in a large bowl. Coat the mix with the dressing and place in the refrigerator to marinate.

Over low heat, warm the Kamut flour tortillas in a large pan till supple. Season with sea salt and cayenne pepper. Fill the tortillas with the salad and roll it up. Serve and enjoy.

## Mushroom, Vegan Cheese, Besides Almond Risotto

### Ingredients

- Cayenne Pepper

- 1½ Cups of Arborio Rice

- 1½ Tablespoons of Butter

- 8 Ounce of Baby Bella Mushrooms (Sliced)

- 2 Tablespoon Sliced Almonds

- •24 Ounce of Vegetable broth ½ Cup Grated Vegan Cheese

- •Sea Salt

<u>Preparations</u>

Pour the vegetable broth into a pan and let it simmer over low heat. Make the heat medium and add a pot over it; then add butter into the pot to melt. Add the already cooked rice and let it cook slowly. Let it cook till its color changes to something off-white. Stir frequently.

Add the vegan broth over the rice and cook over low heat.

Put some butter in a skillet over medium heat, add your mushroom in the melted butter. Season with cayenne pepper and sea salt to taste. Let the mushroom sauté until. Keep in a warm bowl.

With a wooden spoon, keep turning the rice. When the former broth has been absorbed in the rice, add more broth to cover the rice and allow to cook some more.

Toast the almonds at 350 degrees in the oven till brown. When done, place aside. You may need to add more broth to cook properly but not get mushy.

When rice is cooked well, add mushrooms and cheese. Season with sea salt and cayenne pepper. Then serve and top with the toasted almonds, enjoy.

## Asian Sesame Dressing and Noodles
### Ingredients

• 2 Tablespoons of Sesame Butter (Tahini)

• ½ Teaspoon of Lemon

• 1 Freshly Squeezed Clove Garlic (Minced)

• 1 Tablespoon of Raw Sesame Seeds (Toppings)

• 1 Scallion (Chopped)

• Red Bell Pepper and Carrot (Sliced)

• Asian Sesame Dressing

• 2 Teaspoons Gluten-Free Tamari

• ½ Teaspoon of Liquid Coconut Nectar (Coconut Secrets Brand)

### Preparations

You can use either Kelp or zucchini or Kelp noodles. If you are using kelp noodles, soak in warm water for 10 mins. On the other hand, if you are using zucchini noodles, make it with a spiralizer or vegetable peeler.

Take a bowl and add all the dressing ingredients and mix well with a spoon. After this, add the Asian sesame dressing to the noodle and scallion and mix.

You can garnish with sesame seeds and enjoy.

## Fat-Free Peach Muffins
### Ingredients

• 2 Large Peaches about 2 Cups (Chopped)

• 1½ Teaspoons of Mashed Burro Banana

• 1 Tablespoon of Agave Syrup

• 2 Cups of Spelt Flour

• ¼ Teaspoon Salt

• 2 Tablespoons of Warm Spring Water

• 2 Teaspoon of Key Lime Juice

• 1¼ Cups of Homemade Walnut Milk

• 2 Tablespoons of Chopped Walnuts

• ½ Cup of Date Sugar

## Preparations

Begin by setting preheating your oven to 400 °F. Rub a small quantity of grapeseed oil on your muffin pan. Get your peaches and peel off the skin. Add key lime juice, walnut milk, and burro banana and mix properly. Get a bowl, add a pinch of sea salt, date sugar, and flour and mix properly.

Add the liquid ingredients into the mix and stir till a fine batter. Fold the peaches well and distribute well on top of the batter. Fill the muffin to ½ inch of the top, and smoothen the top of the muffin. If you like, sprinkle some chopped walnuts on top. Bake for about 20 mins. You can keep checking with the toothpick, once the toothpick comes out clean, then it is ready. Let the muffins cool down, then serve.

## Younger For Life Mushroom Risotto
## Ingredients

• Sea Salt to taste

• 4 Cups of Homemade Vegetable Broth (choose from Dr. Sebi's approved vegetables)

• 2 Cups of wild Rice

- 4 Mushrooms

- Cayenne Pepper to taste

- 1 Tablespoon Grapeseed Oil

## Preparations

Over medium heat, add your grapeseed oil into a big pot. Put in your onions and mushrooms in the pot and let it cook till the mushrooms are brown and the liquid has reduced drastically. Stir and mix occasionally stir.

Add your cooked rice and let it boil for a minute. Put in the broth, cayenne pepper, sea salt, and then cover the pot to cook until the rice is soft as desired.

Serve and enjoy.

## Kamut Porridge
### Ingredients

- 1 tablespoon coconut oil

- A cup of Kamut or 7 ounces of Kamut,

- ½ teaspoon sea salt

- 3 ¾ cups of soft-jelly coconut milk or walnut milk

•4 tablespoon agave syrup

Preparations

Blend your Kamut in a blender till just cracked and up to 1¼ cups. Mix the cracked Kamut, walnut, or coconut milk and sea salt in a pan or bowl, stir till completely mixed.

In a pan, heat the mix for 10 mins. Then, boil over high heat and after some seconds, reduce the heat. Stir often till you get your desired consistency.

When out of the heat, add coconut oil or agave syrup to your boiled Kamut mix and stir. Serve and enjoy. You can add fresh fruits if you please.

## Blackened Tempeh by Cajun Vegan Ranch
Ingredients for Cajun vegan

•3 tablespoons of Cajun spice

•½ lemon zest

•2 tablespoons olive oil

•½ sea salt

•I block tempeh

•4 radishes (sliced)

- For blackened tempeh

- 1 scallion (sliced)

- ½ teaspoon paprika and ¼ teaspoon cayenne or ½ Cajun spice.

- 1 avocado (sliced)

- ½ cup vegan ranch dressing

- Sprouts ½ cup onion (optional)


## Preparations

Place all the ingredients for the Cajun dressing in a bowl and stir well, taste till the taste is evident. Add a pot on the heat and pour water and add salt. Add tempeh to water, allow the water to cover it, and cook for 10 mins to reduce its bitterness and make it soft.

Have the tempeh sliced into tiny bits and coat each slice in Cajun spice. Heat oil and put the tempeh and stir till crunchy. Set aside. Take out the sharp kale stem and slice like ribbons.

Take a bowl and put in your kale, drizzle 2 tablespoons of olive oil till well coated. Add a little lemon zest and a pinch of salt.

Give the Kale a soft massage, then add radishes, scallion, avocado, and pickled onions. Pour some Cajun dressing and mix efficiently. Dish and serve like this or warm the salad with blackened tempeh with some sprouts.

## Sebi's Sweet Sunrise Smoothie
### Ingredients

- 1 cup mango

- 1 cup of water

- 1/2 burro banana

- 1 cup raspberries

- 1 Seville orange

### Preparations

Add all the ingredients to a high-powered processor and blend till smooth.

## Cinnamon Apple Quinoa
### Ingredients

- 2 large-sized apples

- 2 teaspoons cinnamon

- 1½ cups water

- Honey

- ½ cup quinoa

## Preparations

Peel the apples and chop them into tiny pieces. Take a pan and add some water to it, add the diced apples and quinoa, and cover. Leave to boil for 25 minutes over low heat.

Then add cinnamon to the boiled mixture and stir properly. Add honey and more of the cinnamon if you please. Serve and enjoy.

## Vegan Tlayudas
### Ingredients

- ½ of 16 ounces cabbage (shredded)

- 4-grain tortillas, each approximately 10 inches wide.

- 1 cup carrots (shredded)

- 4 sliced radishes (optional)

- ¼ cup red onions (sliced)

- ¾ teaspoon sea salt

- ½ cucumber (sliced)

- 2 tablespoons olive oil or its substitutes

- ¼ cup scallion (sliced)

- 3 tablespoon of lemon juice with a little zest

- 1 cup of salt

- Avocado cilantro sauce for saucing

- Coriander and cumin sautéed blacked beans (for garnish)

For avocado cilantro sauce

6 slices of jalapeno

1 perfectly ripped avocado of medium size

1 garlic clove

2 tablespoons of olive oil

¼ cup cilantro

2 tablespoons of lime

¼ teaspoon sea salt

4 tablespoon spring water

Preparations

Heat the oven to about 275 degrees Fahrenheit, put in the tortillas, and toast for 20 minutes or till crispy. Mix the radish, carrots, cabbage, and onion and add salt to taste.

Then add the cilantro, cucumber, and scallion and mix thoroughly. Add a dash of lime juice and oil with a little lemon zest. Let it simmer a bit in the bowl.

Make the avocado sauce by mixing all the unlisted ingredients and combine till very smooth, then put in a bowl.

Heat the sautéed beans and use some water and a fork to loosen it up. Season with salt, cumin, and coriander.

Place some beans on the crisp tortilla and add coles slaw.

Use a spoon to spread the avocado sauce on the slaw. Lastly, garnish with a lime wedge, shallot, and pickled onions. Serve and enjoy.

## Vegetarian Biryani
### Ingredients

• 2 tablespoons of olive oil

• 3 rough chopped garlic

• 1 tablespoon coriander

• 1 teaspoon cinnamon

• ½ teaspoon cardamom or 3 mashed cardamom pods

• 1 bay leaf

• 2 cups rinsed basmati rice

• ¼ cup chopped parsley and cashew nuts (for garnishing)

• ½ cup raisins

• 1 large onion (sliced)

• 2 cups chopped veggies (including carrots and zucchini)

- 1 tablespoon chopped ginger

- 1 tablespoon cumin

- 1 teaspoon of chili powder

- ½ teaspoon turmeric

- ¾ cup rinsed and drained chickpeas

Preparations

Take a pan and add some oil and heat in medium heat, then add the onion. Sauté onion till tender. Add your vegetables, ginger, and garlic for about 5 mins.

Take out a cup of this mixture and keep it for later. Then add the bay leaf and other spices and stir for about one minute and then add the basmati rice and sauté for a minute.

Add the raisin, chickpeas, and the cup of veggies you set aside earlier.

Heat to low, cover the pot with a dishtowel, and cover to tighten the seal and keep the steam locked in. Over low heat, cook for about 30 minutes till the rice soak up the entire liquid and turn out the fire.

Open the pot later, top with cilantro and cashew. Food is ready.

## Broccoli Soup
### Ingredients

1 zucchini (1 cup of chopped zucchini)

½ onion (chopped)

6 cup broccoli florets

2 cups vegetable broth

1 or 2 cups almond milk

2 tablespoons lemon juice

1 tablespoon of olive oil

2 carrots (1 cup of chopped carrots)

2 garlic cloves (minced)

½ cup raw cashew nuts

2 cups of Springwater

1 cup nutritional yeast

½ tablespoon sea salt and pepper

## Preparations

Pour olive oil into a skillet and heat it. Then add zucchini, onion, carrots, and garlic to the hot olive oil and cook till the garlic is aromatic. Put in pepper and salt to season.

Add vegetable broth, broccoli, raw cashews, and water. Reduce the heat to low, then put the mixture into a deep pot and allow to simmer for about 20 mins. Then turn off the heat and let it cool down.

Transfer the mixture to a blender and blend. Pour back all the blended mix into the pot and put yeast, lemon juice, and almond milk and mix well.

Add sea salt and pepper for taste. Serve your soup and enjoy.


## Heap of Chickpea Avocado Salad Sandwich
## Ingredients

- 1 ripe avocado

- ¼ cup of cranberries (dried)

- 4 slices of bread (whole grain)

- 1 teaspoon of sea salt and pepper

- 2 teaspoons of fresh lemon juice

- Red onion or spinach for garnish (optional)

- 2 cups of rinsed and drained chickpea

## Preparations

Mash the chickpeas in a bowl with a fork, add avocado and continue to mash till the mixture is smooth. Then add the cranberries and lemon juice and stir. Season with salt and pepper.

Put the dish in the refrigerator for 2 days to marinate.

Serve by toasting your bread, and then spread chickpea avocado on it. Garnish with either red onion or spinach (optional). Place another slice of toasted bread on top. Enjoy your lunch.

## Whole Roasted Cauliflower with Tahini Sauce

### Ingredients

Mint and or parsley for garnishing

1 tablespoon zaatar or cumin or dukkah spice

1 cup of spring water

1 whole cauliflower

2 tablespoons olive oil (share into two parts)

Tahini sauce (1 batch)

1 tablespoon sea salt

## Preparations

Heat up the oven to roughly 425 degrees Fahrenheit and get the cauliflower ready by cutting off the bottom. The trimming will help to give it balance to stand, now add the prepared cauliflower in a pan and drizzle a tablespoon of olive oil over it, season with salt to taste and spice.

Completely seal the pan with a foil and allow to bake for about 55 minutes. Open the pan carefully and add more oil over it and bake for another 30 minutes or when gold.

Top with fresh herbs; parsley or mint and drizzle the whole dish with tahini sauce or in portions when served.

## Ginger and Turmeric Carrot Soup
### Ingredients

1 can of coconut milk

1 cup of chopped butternut squash or more carrots (if butternut is unavailable)

1 cleaned sliced leek

3 cups of chopped carrots

2 garlic (minced)

1 tablespoon of grated ginger

Sea salt and pepper

1 tablespoon of oil (olive or coconut)

1 cup of chopped fennel

1 tablespoon turmeric powder

3 cups vegetable broth with low sodium

## Preparations

Preheat oil with an oven or a saucepan. Add fennel, carrots, leeks, and squash to the heated oil, let it fry for 4 minutes till soft. Then add garlic, pepper, ginger, turmeric, and sea salt, allow to fry for some time.

Take this mix and pour into a bigger pot, then add coconut milk and broth and turn properly, leave to boil for 20 minutes over low heat.

Turn off the heat and let it cool. When cool, pour into a blender and blend till creamy. Taste and add more seasoning if need be.

# Vegan Pecan Apple Chickpea Salad Wraps

## Ingredients

- 1/3 cup of dried tart cherries

- ¼ cup of chopped green onions

- 1 cup of diced apples

- 1 celery stalk

- 1 cup of rinsed chickpeas

- 1/3 cup of raw or toasted pecans

- 2 tablespoons of chopped parsley leaf

## For dressing

- 2 teaspoons of maple syrup

- ¼ teaspoon of garlic powder

- ¼ teaspoon of sea salt

- 3 tablespoons of warm spring water

- 3 tablespoons of tahini

- 1 teaspoon Dijon mustard

- 1 teaspoon apple cider vinegar

- Ground black pepper

For wrapping

- 4 cups of organic spinach

- 3 large size spinach tortillas

- ¾ cup of shredded carrots

Preparation

Mash the chickpeas in a bowl with a fork to be rough, add chopped pecans, parsley, diced apples, green onions, and tart cherries, and all to the bowl ill mixture is smooth.

In another bowl prepare the dressing by adding all the ingredients listed for the purpose and mixing till creamy. Feel free to add more water for your desired consistency.

You can now add the dressing to the chickpea salad bowl and stir to properly coat. You can add more spice if needed.

Spread out the spinach wrap and spread a cup of organic spinach with ¼ cup of shredded carrots.

Add chickpea salad mix and roll up wrap tightly and tuck in at both ends. Repeat this method for the number of wraps you intend to do.

# Date Night Vegan Alfredo

## Ingredients

- ½ teaspoon miso paste (white)

- ½ teaspoon sea salt

- 1 tablespoon nutritional yeast

- 1 teaspoon nutmeg

- 1 cup veggie broth (or water)

- 5 ounces' dry spelt pasta

- 4 garlic cloves

- 1 cup fresh peas

- ½ onion (white preferably)

- 8 ounces of sautéed or smoked mushrooms

- ½ cup raw cashew nuts or hemp seeds

- Chili flakes, lemon zest, pepper, and parsley for garnishing

- Olive oil (2 tablespoons)

## Preparations

Cook pasta in salted water. To make the sauce, heat the olive over low heat and add onions and garlic to the sauté till it is golden. Put out the heat and let it cool. When cool, pour in a blender with the vegetable broth, yeast, cashew nuts, salt, and miso. This will blend till creamy.

If you are using sautéed mushrooms; heat the oil in a pan and then add mushrooms and season with salt. Let it fry till the mushroom gets soft. Take out the water from the cooked pasta. Take a big-sized pan and pour the pasta and sauce into it and stir well. Add the mushrooms and mix well. Put in the lemon zest, chill flakes, pepper, and chopped parsley to garnish this lovely dish.

Serve and enjoy.

## Pumpkin Steel Cut Oats
### Ingredients

• 1 teaspoon pumpkin pie spice

• 1 tablespoon of coconut oil

• ¼ teaspoon sea salt

• ½ cup of pumpkin puree

- ½ cup of caramelized pecans

- 3 cups almond milk

- 2 tablespoons of coconut oil

- ¾ cup of steel-cut oats

- Extra almond milk for drizzling and pecans (optional)

- ¼ cup of coconut sugar (divided into 2 portions)

## Preparations

Get a pan and add the oats and almond milk and boil. Add pumpkin, vegan butter, coconut sugar, sea salt, and pumpkin spice, and stir well till all is blended properly.

Add caramelized pecans and allow to cook till the dish caramelizes. Your food is ready. Serve the oats and add more almond milk and pecans if you like.

## Tofu Burger
### Ingredients for a tofu burger

- 400g of tofu

- 1 tablespoon of pepper and sea salt

- Breadcrumbs 100g

- 2 tablespoons of oil (either olive or coconut)

## Ingredients for sauce

- 1 cup of ground fresh tomatoes

- Red wine

- 3 tablespoons of tamari

- 1 sliced onion

- 1 teaspoon apple cider vinegar

- 1 tablespoon of olive oil

- 1 tablespoon of sea salt and pepper

## For serving

Burger buns, tomatoes, or salad lettuce

## Preparations for burgers

Use your hands to mash the tofu and place in a blender and blend till fine. Add salt, breadcrumbs, and pepper to a bowl and mix lightly with your hands.

Flatten out the patties to make 6 burgers out of them. Put oil in a pan and heat it up, then place tofu patties in the hot oil. Flip both sides until they turn golden.

Preparations for sauce

Note, this sauce can be prepared alongside the burgers.

Heat some oil, add onion and sauté for 5 minutes. Pour red wine and cook till the wine evaporates. After add tamari, tomato, date syrup, vinegar, pepper, and salt.

Allow to boil over low heat for 15 mins. Add more seasoning if need be.

Serve with salad and sauce on the burger.

## Oaxacan Bowl
Ingredients

- ½ cup pecans

- 1 teaspoon sea salt

- 1 teaspoon ground chipotle

- ½ red onion

- 2 teaspoons of cumin

- 1 medium-size sweet potato or yam (diced into little cubes with skin on it)

- 8 baby bell peppers or 1 regular sized red pepper (sliced)

- 2 teaspoons maple syrup

- Avocado, scallion, cilantro, for garnishing

- Fresh black beans sautéed with seasoning

Ingredients for quick cabbage slaw

- 1 tablespoon lemon juice

- 1 tablespoon olive oil

- ¼ cup of either chopped cilantro or scallion or both

- A quarter of shredded red cabbage (shredded)

- 1 teaspoon coriander

- 1 teaspoon sea salt

Preparation

Heat up the oven to 400 degrees Fahrenheit. Mix the cumin, chipotle, and salt in a bowl. Take a lined pan and add some onions, sweet potato, and pepper. Drizzle some oil over it and add little spices and toss to coat well.

Put the pan in the oven for about 30 mins and flip in 10 mins. Ready another lined sheet pan and put your pecan, a tablespoon of mixed spice, and maple syrup and toss well.

Put in the oven till it turns golden. Flip as soon as you take it down so the nuts will easily loosen up.

Heat the earlier sautéed seasoned beans. Make slaw by finely chopping cabbage and pour in a bowl with the leftover ingredients. Mix and taste, add salt and lime as desired.

Slice the avocado and separate beans into 3 bowls. Add veggies, avocado, and slaw to each bowl. Serve with avocado sauce if you like.

## Spelt Granola

## Ingredients

2 tablespoons of avocado oil

2 cups spelt flakes

½ cup chopped walnuts

¼ cup hemp, sesame seeds, and pumpkin

½ cup chopped dry seeded fruit

4 tablespoon of agave syrup

Sea salt

½ coconut flakes (dried)

## Preparations

Heat up the oven to 300 degrees Fahrenheit. Take a bowl and place all the ingredients and stir. Keep stirring till the dried condiments are soaked in the oil, agave syrup, and sea salt.

When the mixture is sticky and thick, place it into the preheated oven for 10 mins. Serve and enjoy.

## Roasted Rainbow Vegetable Bowl

## Ingredients

½ large size sweet potato (sliced round with skin on)

2 large carrots (half sliced)

4 medium yellow or red potato

4 radishes

2 tablespoons of coconut or avocado oil

1 sliced beet

1 teaspoon curry powder

1 cup of sliced cabbage

1 sliced red pepper

½ teaspoon of sea salt

1 cup of chopped broccoli

2 cups of chopped organic kale or collard

For toppings

2 tablespoons of tahini

3 tablespoons of lemon juice

2 tablespoons of hemp seeds

½ avocado (optional)

Preparations

Preheat oven to 200 degrees Celsius. Place 2 baking pans with paper. Add sweet potatoes, carrots, radishes, potatoes, and beet to one pan, drizzle with a tablespoon of oil or water. Add curry powder and salt to taste and stir well. Bake in the preheated oven for 25 mins.

Put broccolini, cabbage, and pepper in the other pan and drizzle with a tablespoon of oil or water. Also, season with curry powder and salt and stir. Place in the oven to bake for 15 mins. Add the kale and collard greens to the pan and roast till it looks bright green.

Serve and enjoy, you can garnish with avocado, and season with tahini, salt, lemon juice, and hemp seeds.

## Spelt Roti

### Ingredients

- 1 teaspoon sea salt

- 1 cup spelt flour

- Springwater

- 2 teaspoon grapeseed oil

### Directions

Mix all ingredients in a big bowl. The outcome will look like a soft spongy-like dough. Let it sit for 30 mins, then heat a pan with oil. Cut dough into rolls of 12 balls and dip balls into the spelt flour each after the other. Roll thin and flat and form a circular roti. Put the roti in a hot dry pan, once the roti begins to bubble, flip and remove the roti when you notice it bubbling again.

# Vegan Fried Rice Topped with Tofu

## Ingredients

- 1 cup of brown rice

- 1 cup of tofu

- 4 garlic cloves

- ½ cup of peas

- 1 cup of green chopped onion

- ½ cup of diced carrot

## For sauce

- 2 teaspoon of chili sauce

- 1 teaspoon of sesame oil or avocado oil (optional)

- 3 teaspoons of tamari

- 1 tablespoon of peanut butter

- 3 tablespoons of maple syrup or honey

- 1 minced garlic clove

## Preparations

Heat the oven to 204 degrees Celsius and use a nonstick pan or spray a pan with a non-stick spray inside.

Wrap tofu with an absorptive cloth and drain water by placing it under a heavy object.

When the oven is ready and the tofu drained, cut into cubes and put in a pan. Leave in the oven till brown.

Put rice in a big pot and fill it with about 12 cups of water. Boil on high heat for 30 mins. Strain out water for 10 seconds and pour rice back into pot and cover with foil to steam for 10 mins - don't forget to take down from the heat.

Preparations for sauce

Put all the ingredients for the sauce and blend. Add tamari, flavor, peanut butter, honey, as desired.

Add sauce to complete baking tofu for 5 minutes and stir frequently.

Take a big skillet and scoop the tofu into the pan without the sauce. Roast until all the sides are golden. Take out from the pan and set it aside, do this process for the rest. Sauté carrots, green onions, peas, and garlic in a hot skillet. Stir well and season with tamari or soy sauce.

Add the rice, tofu, and leftover sauce and stir well. Over medium heat, leave to cook for 4 mins. Serve with cashew or roasted peanuts.

## Instantaneous Pot Mujadara
## Ingredients

- •1 cup brown basmati rice

- •1½ tablespoons of olive oil

- •1 cup of brown lentils

- •3 shallots or 1 red onion (sliced)

- •2 teaspoons cumin

- •4 garlic cloves (roughly chopped)

- •1 teaspoon coriander

- •½ teaspoon cinnamon

- •1 teaspoon of a mix of allspice

- •½ teaspoon of ground ginger

- •1 teaspoon dried parsley or mint

- 1½ teaspoons sea salt

- 3 cups spring water

- 1 teaspoon lemon zest

- Carrots, yogurt, sprouts, roasted veggies for garnishing (optional)

## Preparations

In a bowl, cover lentils with hot spring water and let them soak. Put a pot to sauté. Add oil and shallots over low heat till they are a bit caramelized. Take half of this a place in a small bowl to be used for later. Add garlic to the other half in the pan and sauté for another 2 minutes, then add zest, salt, water, and other spices and stir. Add the earlier drained lentils and rinsed rice to the pot.

Cover the pot and cook for about 10 mins. Garnish with whatever you desire; caramelized shallots, yogurt, avocado, roasted vegetables, parsley, a drizzle of oil, or mint.

## Brazil Nut and Banana Cookies

### Ingredients

- 2 bananas (to be mashed)

- 1 ½ teaspoons cinnamon (ground)

- Scottish oats 200g (reserve ¼ of the oats)

- Buckwheat flour 30g )

- 1½ tablespoons of flax seeds

- 3 tablespoons sunflower seeds

- A handful of chopped brazil nuts

- 3 tablespoons maple syrup

- 200ml olive oil or sunflower oil

- 1 teaspoon baking soda

- 1 teaspoon of almond extract

Preparations

Heat the oven to 180 degrees Celsius. Add all condiments into a shallow bowl and mix till it forms a smooth dough.

Add oats and stir. Bake for 10 mins if you like your cookies sift. If you want a crispier cookie, leave for another 4 mins. Bring out the cookies from the oven and let them cool off. Breakfast is served.

# Vegan Corn Chowder

## Ingredients

- 2 tablespoons olive oil

- 1 diced red pepper

- ½ white diced onion

- 2 stalks of diced celery

- 2 diced potatoes

- 3 cups of fresh corn kernels

- 3 cups of veggie stock

- 1 cup of coconut milk

- 1 teaspoon of salt

- ½ teaspoon of black pepper

- 2 tablespoons of chopped chives

## Preparations

Get a pan and add olive oil to it, heat over medium heat. Put in onions, celery, and pepper and stir for 5 mins. Add the rest of the condiments asides the 1 cup of corn and chives. Cook till potatoes are soft then take down the pot and leave to cool. When cold, pour into a blender or food processor and blend as desired. Put the soup back in the pot and the leftover corn kernels and turn. Let the soup simmer for 10 mins and then add chives and turn well. Your food is ready, serve and enjoy.

## Veggie Lo Mein!
### Ingredients for lo Mein sauce

•3 tablespoons of soy sauce

•2 tablespoons of Chinese cooking wine

•2 teaspoons sesame oil

•1 teaspoon honey (or sugar or maple syrup)

•1 teaspoon of white pepper

•1 teaspoon of sriracha

### Ingredient for lo Mein fry

•½ sliced onion

•2 tablespoons of coconut or peanut oil

•2 cups of sliced mushrooms

•3 garlic cloves

•1 teaspoon minced ginger

- ½ of sliced bell pepper

- 1 cup carrots

- 1 cup of snow peas

- 1 cup of shredded cabbage

- Slice scallions for garnishing

## Preparations

Prepare noodles in salted water. Get a bowl and add all the condiments for lo Mein sauce and mix. Get all the veggies ready.

Heat the coconut oil in a pan and sauté mushrooms and onion for 5 minutes, stirring frequently. Under medium heat, add the ginger and garlic for another 2 mins. Add the pepper, cabbage, carrots, and peas. Stir till soft and crisp.

Toss in the drained noodle and mix well. Add sauce and stir properly for 2 mins, if too dry add some water.

Serve and garnish with scallions.

## Spelt Pasta
## Ingredients

3 to 6 tablespoons of spring water

½ teaspoon sea salt

2½ cups of whole spelt flour

2 tablespoons olive oil

Directions

Make a pile of spelt flour and scatter the sea salt on top. Make a hole in the middle and pour the mixture of oil and 3 tablespoons of water.

Knead flour gently and add a tablespoon of water per time. Make the dough smooth and flexible by kneading for 10 mins. Cut dough in form of little balls and cover. Leave it at room temperature for an hour.

Take one-fourth of the dough and flatten out the shape and roll the dough with the help of a pasta machine. Cut dough in accordant to the size of noodles needed and allow the pasta to cool and form. Do the same process to the leftover dough.

Get a hollow pot and add salted water to cook the pasta. Once you add the pasta, stir so it doesn't begin to stick. Boil till pasta is tender.

# Sun-Dried Tomato Alfredo

## Ingredients

- ¼ cup of chopped fresh basil

- Olive oil (1 tablespoon)

- 1 tablespoon of oregano

- 2 tablespoons of arrowroot flour

- 2 tablespoons of tomato paste

- ½ cup of dried tomatoes

- ¼ cup vegan parmesan

- 3 garlic cloves (broken)

- 1 pound of any shape chickpea pasta

- 1½ cups of almond milk

## Directions

Cook pasta (see recipe and directions above).

Put a skillet with oil on medium heat and sauté some garlic for about a minute, then add dried tomatoes (half portion), oregano, and arrowroot. Stir properly.

Add almond milk on low heat and leave to thicken a bit. Add tomato paste and vegan Parmesan and stir. Let the sauce cool off and then transfer to a blender and blend till creamy. Place the sauce in a pan and add your pasta gently while stirring.

Put the leftover dried tomatoes and basil or Parmesan to garnish. Your meal is ready.

## Ecstatic Smoothie
### Ingredients

¼ Pitted Avocado

1 Chopped Pear

1 Ounce of Blueberries

1 Cup of Water

¼ Cup of Cooked Quinoa

### Preparation

First, wash the ingredients properly. Add all the condiments into a fast blender or food processor and blend till smooth. Then your smoothie is ready, take a glass cup and serve yourself. Enjoy.

## Mixed Berry Smoothie
### Ingredients

½ cup sliced fresh raspberries

½ cup of fresh sliced strawberries

¼ cup of yellow banana

1 cup of fresh blueberries

1 tablespoon raw hemp seed

1 teaspoon maple syrup

2 teaspoons sea moss gel or powder

## Preparation

Keep some berries away for garnish later. Add banana and berries to a blender and blend till smooth.

Transfer inside a bowl and garnish with the reserved berries and hemp seeds. Put some maple syrup over the top if you wish.

## Peanut Spinach Udon
### Ingredients

- ½ tablespoon peanut butter

- 1 tablespoon sesame oil

- 1 tablespoon soy sauce

- ½ tablespoon of lime juice

- 1 minced garlic clove

- 1 bundle udon

- 1½ cups of baby spinach

- 2 sliced green onion

- ½ teaspoon of ginger

- ½ tablespoon honey

- 1 tablespoon sesame seeds for garnish

Preparations

Make the Udon noodles. Prepare the spinach by putting all condiments, begin with the baby spinach. Add more seasoning as desired. When the pasta is cooked, drain out and set aside. Put an empty pot on the cooker and add ½ tablespoon of green onions and sliced spinach. Turn in the noodles and let them cook for 3 minutes. Don't forget to turn gently in the sauce till it mixes properly. Add more soy sauce if you wish. Garnish with sesame seeds and green onions.

# Roasted Portobello Mushrooms with Walnut Coffee Sauce

## Ingredients

- 1 tablespoon balsamic vinegar

- 4 big portobello mushrooms

- 1 teaspoon of sea salt and pepper

## Ingredients for walnut sauce

- 3 tablespoons olive oil

- 2 roughly diced large shallots

- 1 cup raw walnut

- 4 roughly diced garlic cloves

- ½ teaspoon sea salt

- ½ teaspoon miso

- 1 teaspoon balsamic

- Green herbs

- truffle oil

- thyme

•pomegranate seeds for topping

Preparations

Heat up the oven to 400 degrees Fahrenheit. Mix vinegar with oil. Make use of the brush to touch both sides of the Portobello and add salt and pepper. Flip the gill side down on a lined pan and bake for about 25 minutes. Then wrap in foil till it is ready to be used.

Make the sauce by heating the oil, add garlic and shallots and cook till soft. Toss in walnuts to cook for 2 mins. Turn it off and let it cool. Add salt, balsamic, miso paste, and pepper and blend till smooth.

Put the sauce back in the pan and heat up. Place cooked or sliced portabellas on the walnut sauce to serve.

## Brain-Boosting Smoothie
Ingredients

•½ Cup of Burro Banana

•A cup of stress/nerve relieving herbal tea on Dr. Sebi's approved list

•½ Cup of Blueberries

- ½ Tablespoon of Agave Syrup or Date Sugar

- ½ Cup of Raspberries

## Preparation

Boil a cup of refined water. Take half a tablespoon for the one cup of the stress/nerve-relieving herbal tea and add to the boiling water. Let boil for 15 mins and drain and allow to cool off. When cold, turn the ingredients into the blender and put the cold tea, and blend at high speed. Pour in a cup and enjoy.

## Basil Avocado Pasta Salad

## Ingredients

- 1 Teaspoon of Agave Syrup

- 1 Pint of Halved Cherry Tomatoes

- 1 Tablespoon of Key Lime Juice

- 1 Chopped Avocado

- ¼ Cup of Olive Oil

- 1 Cup of Chopped Fresh Basil

- 4 Cups of Cooked Spelt Pasta

## Preparations

Add the cooked pasta to a large bowl. Add the tomatoes, basil, avocado, and then the pasta and mix properly.

Prepare the dressing in a little bowl by mixing the oil, agave syrup, lime juice, and salt, then add the pasta and stir well.

## Szechuan Tofu and Veggies
## Ingredients

•4 ounces of sliced mushrooms

•½ sliced onion

•1 cup shredded carrots

•½ sliced red pepper

•2 tablespoons olive oil

•1 cup green beans or asparagus

•1 teaspoon sea salt and pepper

•Scallion, chili flake, and sesame seeds for topping

•8 ounces of patted dry tofu

•¼ cup Szechuan sauce

•2 cups of shredded cabbage

## Preparations

Over medium heat, add olive oil to a pan and heat, then add onions, mushrooms and leave for some. Keep stirring.

Add other vegetables and turn down the heat. Sauté for 5 minutes then add a quarter cup of Szechuan sauce till you get the taste you want. Cook for till it becomes thick.

Add crispy tofu for about 1 min and turn off the heat.

Serve with sprinkles of sesame seeds and scallions and sesame seeds over the rice or noodles.

## Triple Berry Smoothie
### Ingredients

- ½ Cup of Strawberries

- ½ Cup of Raspberry

- 1 Burro Banana

- 1 Cup of Water

- ½ Cup of Blueberries

- Agave Syrup

## Preparations

Wash and clean the fruits. Pour all ingredients into a blender and blend well. Serve and drink the smoothie.

## Dandelion Strawberry Salad
## Ingredients

- 10 Ripe Sliced Strawberries

- 4 Cups of Dandelions

- 2 Tablespoons of Grapeseed Oil

- 1 Medium Sliced Red Onion

- 2 Tablespoons of Key Lime Juice

- Sea Salt

## Preparations

Add grapeseed oil to a pan and fry the diced onions in a pan till golden.

Fry the sliced onions in a frying pan with grapeseed oil until it turns brown. Slice the dandelion greens into small bits and set them aside. In a small bowl, mix the diced strawberries with key lime juice.

Put the remaining key lime juice on the onions before it gets golden and leave to cook till thick. Add and mix all ingredients in a salad bowl, add salt to taste.

## Quinoa Pasta with Creamy Carrot Miso Sauce

### Ingredients

- 1 garlic clove

- 10 ounces' quinoa pasta cooked in sea salted water

- 2 roughly chopped shallots or onions

- ½ cup parsley or tender carrot tops

- 2 tablespoons olive oil

- ¼ cup raw cashew nuts

- 2 cups spring water

- 2 full cups of sliced medium carrots

- ¼ tablespoon sea salt

- ¼ teaspoon pepper

- 6 chopped garlic cloves

- 1 tablespoon lemon zest

- 3 tablespoons white miso paste

## Preparations

Prepare pasta with salted water. Heat the oil over medium heat. Then add garlic and shallot and let it cook till golden. Stir properly, add carrots, cashew nut, pepper, salt, and water. Turn and cover to boil, reduce the heat to steam slightly till carrot is soft.

Put 3 tsp. of Miso and turn off the heat and leave to cool for about 10 mins. Pour into a blender and cover closely with a towel. Later blend till creamy. Then drain pasta well and turn in the sauce. Mix well and season properly. Sprinkle bread crumbs over the food when served.

## Alkaline Mineral Smoothie
### Ingredients

- ½ Large Seed Papaya

- 1 Tablespoon of Bromide Plus Powder

- 2 Burro Banana

- Juice of half a key lime

- 1 Cup of Fresh Spring Water

- 4-5 Date Sugar

Preparations

Wash and clean the fruits, in a high-speed blender, add the water and the fruits. Blend the ingredients till smooth. Serve in a glass cup and enjoy.

## Stewed Okra and Tomatoes

Ingredients

- 1 Cup of Cherry Tomatoes

- 1 Medium Sized Onion

- ½ Cup of Fresh Spring Water

- 1 Tablespoon of Avocado Oil

- Cayenne Pepper and Sea Salt

- 2 Cups of Fresh Okra

Preparations

Peel the onions and cherry tomatoes and slice them. Add avocado oil to a skillet and then add the onions and fry till translucent. Put in the spring water and okra, let it cook on low heat for about 10 mins. Add cherry tomatoes and let cook for 20 mins. Then add sea salt and pepper.

# Supper Frankie's

## Ingredients

- 1 tablespoon coriander

- ¾ teaspoon sea salt

- 1 tablespoon of coconut oil or olive oil

- 2 teaspoons of yellow curry powder

- 1 teaspoon fennel seed or coriander seed (optional)

- Chickpea and roasted cauliflower

- 1 teaspoon of granulated garlic or onion powder

- 1 head cauliflower (chopped)

- 2 tablespoons of olive oil

- 1 cup of rinse and properly drained chickpeas

- 1½ teaspoon sea salt

- 1 tablespoon cumin

- 16 ounces' potatoes (reserve ¼)

## Ingredients for burrito

- 4 large grain tortillas

- 1 cup of baby spinach

- 2 tablespoons of cilantro mint chutney

- 2 tablespoons of pickled onions

## Preparations

Heat up the oven to about 425 degrees Fahrenheit. cut potatoes and put them in a pot of water. Then cover for the potatoes to simmer till very soft. Cut the cauliflower into tiny pieces and put it on a corner of a parchment-lined pan.

Put the chickpeas on a side of the pan, drizzle oil on cauliflower and chickpea, then season with salt and spices.

Toss the sides to coat well. Preheat oven for 25 minutes, put it in after 10 mins. Prepare cilantro mint chutney and pickled onions in a jar (it's best to make this earlier).

Take out the potatoes once very soft, drain out the hot water but leave aside a cup of water. Put the potatoes into a large pot and mash, keep adding hot water little by little as desired.

Add oil, spices, and salt, mix till well blended. Add water till it becomes a spreadable mash. Taste to make sure the seasoning and spice are as desired. Cover and leave warm. When the vegetables are ready, warm the tortillas and spread them evenly with curried potatoes, chickpeas, and cauliflowers.

Add a handful of spinach leaves, cilantro mint chutney, and onions, and roll up the burrito. Your food is ready.

## Hale and Hearty Fried Rice
### Ingredients

•1 Cup of Wild Rice or Quinoa

•½ Cup of Mushrooms

•½ Cup of Bell Peppers

•½ Cup of Zucchini

•¼ Onion

•1 Tablespoon of Grapeseed Oil

•Cayenne Pepper and Sea Salt to taste

### Preparations

Wash the rice and parboil it well. Chop the mushroom, bell pepper, onion, and zucchini. Put some grapeseed oil in a frying pan and heat up, then add onions and sauté till golden.

Add all the sliced veggies and let it cook till soft. Put your cooked rice and cook till brown. Serve and enjoy.

# Conclusion

In conclusion, this cookbook is much more than a mere collection of recipes; it's a comprehensive guide to a rejuvenated, healthier, and more youthful you. By focusing on anti-inflammatory foods, antioxidants, low glycemic ingredients, and stress-reducing meals, each recipe is crafted to combat the Four Horsemen of Aging effectively.

These aren't just dishes; they're a blend of science and art, designed to nourish your body at the deepest levels. If you incorporate these carefully prepared recipes into your diet, you are not just feeding your body; you are nurturing it.

This is not merely about eating; it's about living a life filled with vitality and youthfulness. Embrace these recipes, and you'll find yourself on a path to "Younger for Life," where every meal is a step towards lasting health and rejuvenation.

# Recommendation

Younger For Life – A Step-By Step Guide to reversing the effects of aging By Dr. Anthony Youn

Link>>   https://www.amazon.com/Younger-Life-Great-Science-Autojuvenation/dp/1335007873